I0411721

THE PROGRESSIVE BARBER

A BOOK FOR THE APPRENTICE
AND FOR THE BARBER

DESCRIBING THE

ANATOMY AND PHYSIOLOGY OF THE SKIN

DISEASES OF THE SKIN

THAT ARE OF SPECIAL INTEREST TO THE
BARBER

AND

THE USE OF ANTISEPTICS

AND THEIR VALUE

By
ARNOLD DREXEL, M. D.
MILWAUKEE,
WIS.

PREFACE

The author of this book took special pains to avoid as much as possible, all medical terms that may confuse the apprentice, or the barber. The anatomy and physiology of the skin is described in detail, because references are made to them frequently in the after reading. Only the diseases that are of interest to the barber are mentioned. The treatments for the various diseases mentioned were purposely omitted, because the barber is not allowed by law to treat diseases. Only the most valuable antiseptics are recommended. The reader should not condemn the author on account of the so frequently mentioning of alcohol as an antiseptic or a disinfectant, as he considers it the cleanest, strongest and quickest acting disinfectant, which can be easily employed, that leaves no odor, and does no harm to the barber's instruments.

A. D.

ANATOMY OF THE SKIN

The skin forms the external covering of the whole surface of the body and is in intimate relation with the underlying structures. Its outer surface is not uniform to the eye nor to the touch. The color varies considerably with age, sex, race, and climate, as well as in different localities of the body in the same individual. The dark color of the skin depends upon the presence of a layer, or smaller number of blackish-brown pigment granules in the upper layers of the skin. The thickness greatly differs in different regions, being most pronounced over the palms of the hands and the soles of the feet, least so, over the eyelids and the genitals. On close inspection we will see numerable ridges, furrows, and pores, and the presence of various sized hairs, and on the fingers and toes, the hardened nail formation. The furrows are either long and deep, or short and superficial, dividing the surface into a large number of oblong or lozenge shaped fields. They are mostly found in the flexures of the joints.

The pores are minute depressions, representing the openings of the glands and hair follicles which are situated in the skin.

Grossly speaking, the skin consists of the following three marked layers:

First, the epidermis or outer layer of the skin;

Second, the derma, cutis, corium, true skin or deep layer;

Third, the subcutaneous tissue.

Blood vessels and lymphatics are situated in the derma or true skin, or subcutaneous tissue.

Nerves are situated in all layers, except the outermost layer of the epidermis.

The appendages of the skin are four in number, viz.: sweat glands, sebaceous or oil glands, hair and nails.

5

THE EPIDERMIS

The epidermis, the most external of the layers of the skin, is conveniently divided into four layers; the outermost layer, or stratum corneum, known as the horny layer; below this an ill-defined, shining layer, or stratum lucidum; and beneath this the granular layer, or stratum granulosum; and finally the innermost layer, or mucous layer.

Stratum Corneum.

The stratum corneum, horny layer, or dead layer, is the outermost external portion of the epidermis. Scales are continually thrown off by this layer.

Stratum Lucidum.

This layer is immediately below the horny layer, is of a glistening appearance, narrow and compact.

Stratum Granulosum.

This layer lies below the stratum lucidum. Nothing of importance can be said about it.

Stratum Mucosum.

This layer is the deepest layer of the epidermis, and is of importance. In the lower portion of this layer we find the cells containing the coloring matter, known as pigment, which gives the skin a brownish appearance. In the Caucasian race these are best observed in the regions of the nipples of the breast, the scrotum, the anus and the external female genital organs.

In the colored races we find the pigment in greater amount. Nerves are found running through this layer to the outer layers of the epidermis.

Corium.

The corium, derma, or true skin, is composed of dense interlacing bundles of fibrous connective tissue.

6

It contains blood vessels, nerves, lymphatics, hairs, glands, fat cells, and a varying amount of smooth muscles.

Subcutaneous Tissue.

This layer lies beneath the corium and contains the sweat glands, the deeper lying hair follicles, trunks of blood and lymph-vessels, and nerves.

BLOOD VESSELS

Both the corium and the subcutaneous tissue are liberally supplied with blood. The epidermis has no blood supply, and that is the reason why a superficial cut into the skin does not bleed. This is more perceivable on the palms of the hands and on the soles of the feet, because the horny layer of the epidermis is the thickest at those places. Blood vessels are divided into two classes, arteries and veins. The arteries carry the blood from the heart through the whole body, and the veins return it. The arteries lie deep, whereas the veins lie superficial, and may readily be seen in the skin. Arteries carry fresh blood, that is, blood well supplied with oxygen, and of a bright-red color, whereas veins contain blood minus oxygen, and of a dark-red hue. In former years when cupping and blood letting was practiced to a great extent, the belief was, that the dark blood, drawn from the skin by the cups, or the blood taken direct from the veins, was bad blood, and it was supposed that it was a good thing for the patient that such blood was removed. This, however, is not true, as the venous or darker blood is conducted through the veins to the heart, from there to the lungs, where it is charged with a new supply of oxygen, which brightens the color from a dark-red to a bright-red hue, and des-

7

ignated as arterial blood, and carried from the lungs to the heart and from there is distributed throughout the body. The venous blood by this change has lost all of its formerly supposed unhealthy appearance.

NERVES

Nerves are distributed throuhout the body, including the various glands, muscles, and other structures of the skin. Nerves have the property of transmitting impulses, and control all organs of the body. The main operating center of the nerves is the brain. A nerve may be compared with a wire that transmits an electric current from a battery to a motor, which it sets in motion. All organs of the body are set in motion by a current transmitted to them through the nerves. Nerves also carry impulses of sensation from various parts of the body to the brain or nerve centers. If a nerve is cut, the parts formerly controlled by it will lose all sensation and motor power, and will be designated as being paralyzed.

SWEAT GLANDS

The sweat, or sudoriparous glands, or sweat coils, are small, globular, reddish-yellow bodies, situated in the superficial portion of the subcutaneous tissue, or the deep part of the true skin. From each gland a duct or canal passes through the various parts of the skin, which conducts the sweat to the surface. The sweating, while more or less constant, ordinarily evaporates as rapidly as it is produced, so that its presence is not perceived. If for any reason, however, the function of the glands are increased, as the result of exercise, work, or heat, the secretion is formed much more rapidly, and

8

will be seen on the surface of the skin in the form of drops. The palms, soles, face, neck, and armpits, are favored places for increased sweating. The average amount normally excreted by an adult in twenty-four hours is between two and three pints. The amount can, however, be increased or diminished, depending on various conditions and circumstances, such as heat, cold, clothing, drugs, nervous system, etc.

SEBACEOUS GLANDS

The sebaceous glands, also known as oil glands, are situated in the true skin, formed from the outer root sheath of the hair, and usually in close relation to the hair. In the palms and soles there are no sebaceous glands. Each gland has a canal, through which the oily substance or sebum is conveyed to the hair, and thence to the surface of the skin. In several diseases of the skin these canals are obstructed by the hardening of the sebum. The hardened plugs are generally known as blackheads. When sebaceous glands become very active, the result will be a greasy, shining skin. The sebum acts as a lubricant to the hair, and also keeps the skin soft and pliable. On the scalp, if the secretion is allowed to collect indefinitely, the parts being washed only at long intervals, and only carelessly brushed and combed, it tends to collect in minute, thin, greasy scales, producing a condition called dandruff.

THE HAIR

Hair are horny, rounded formations, arising from the skin. Each hair is divided into two parts: the root, having its seat in the true skin, is implanted in a pouch or follicle, and a shaft, which projects free above the

9

skin. The lower part of the hair or root is thicker than the shaft, and ends in a bulb, known as the hair bulb. A hair consists of a transparent membrane which is outermost, named cuticle, and a central or medullary portion, or marrow. The color of the hair is due to the presence of pigment granules, and diffuse pigment. Gray and light colored hair are without pigment. The hair follicle or hair pouch in which the root of the hair is imbedded, is of connective tissue structure, indirectly connected with a muscle, the arector pili muscle, the function of which is to make the hair stand up straight. A good example of the action of such muscles is seen in the dog, hog and various other animals, when in an angry mood. The hair follicles are supplied with arteries, veins and nerves. The arteries and veins are the nourishing factors of the hair, while the nerves furnish control. Hair are found in all parts of the body surface, except the palms, soles, some parts on the upper surface of the fingers and toes, lips and penis. Hair may be divided into three classes: first, fine, soft or downy hairs, usually seen upon the face, trunk and limbs; second, short, strong hairs, such as the eyebrows, eyelashes, also those in the nose and external ears; third, long hairs, as those of the scalp, beard, armpits and genital regions.

NAILS

Nails are horny, transparent structures, implanted in the skin of the dorsal surfaces of the ends of the fingers and toes. A nail takes the place of the horny layer of the epidermis to which it responds, but differs from it in being harder.

10

THE FUNCTIONS OF THE SKIN

The functions of the skin are manifold, and of great importance. First, the skin furnishes protection for the deeper tissues, muscles, nerves and blood-vessels, from external injuries, by its elasticity and flexibility. The horny layer in being harder than the other layers of the skin, is well adapted for protection from burns, caustics and other injuries; second, the skin is the organ of the sense of touch. We recognize by this, shapes, sizes and other properties of various subjects, heat, cold and injuries; third, absorption. Various substances may be taken up by the skin and carried into the general circulation. Some drugs are absorbed more readily than others, and this fact should be kept in mind when applying poisonous remedies or disinfectants to a large surface of the skin. Watery vapors, oxygen and other gases are absorbed freely; fourth, secretion is a very important function of the skin. The sebaceous and sweat glands perform this function; fifth, the temperature of the body is regulated by the skin, which is of great importance. This regulation takes place by radiation, evaporation and conduction. The horny layer of the skin is a bad conductor of heat, and by this limits too great a loss of heat from the superficial blood vessels. The epidermis also produces a certain amount of pressure upon the blood vessels, preventing their over-filling with blood, and the loss of fluid and heat. In hot weather, or if the skin is exposed to heat, the blood vessels relax and fill up to their greatest capacity, and the result will be sweating. The heat is carried off by the water. If the skin is exposed to cold, the blood vessels shrink, diminishing the amount of blood supply of the skin, which becomes dry, and the giving off of heat is greatly lessened.

11

ABNORMAL CONDITIONS OF THE SKIN
BY WHICH DISEASES ARE RECOGNIZED

It is necessary for the reader to be acquainted with the various lesions of the skin, to enable him to recognize more readily some of the more important diseases with which he may come in contact while shaving, or cutting hair, in order to protect himself as well as his patrons from contagious diseases.

MACULES.—Synonyms—Maculae; Spots; Ger., Flecke.
Macules are discolorations of various tints, shapes and sizes, and level with the skin. Examples of macules are found in the common freckles, which are the result of an excessive amount of pigment in the skin, and in vitiligo where there is a loss of pigment, which gives the spots a clear white appearance. The discolorations of bruises also come under the head of macules.

PAPULES.— Synonyms — Papulae; Pimples; Ger., Knötchen.
Papules are elevations of the skin from the size of a pin's point to a split pea, and not containing fluid. They may occur on any part of the body. The face is most frequently the site of papules.

NODULES.—Synonyms—Nodulae; Ger., Knoten.
Nodules are elevations of the skin ranging from a split pea to a hazelnut in size.

TUMORS.—Synonyms—Tomores; Ger., Knollen; Geschwülste.
Tumors are from a pea upwards in size. They may be soft or hard, and of different constitution, growth, character and termination. They may undergo reaction, and form ulcers. The class of tumors includes

12

diseases as, carbuncles, cancers, leprosy, fatty tumors, wens, and a number of others, of benign or malignant nature.

VESICLES.—Synonyms—Vesiculae; Ger., Bläschen.
Vesicles are elevations of the skin from a pin's point to a small pea in size, and containing fluid. They may be designated as little blisters.

BLEBS.—Synonyms—Bullae; Blisters; Ger., Blasen.
Blebs are elevations of the skin larger than a pea and containing fluid. The distinction from vesicles lies only in the size.

PUSTULES.—Synonyms—Pustulae; Ger., Pusteln.
Pustules, as the name implies, contain pus, and are of various sizes and shapes. Many skin diseases are characterized by pustules. If pustules are found upon the face, the barber should be on the look-out, and disinfect his shaving instruments thoroughly after shaving.

SCALES.—Synonyms—Squamae; Ger., Schuppen.
Scales are exfoliations of a dry nature, from the horny layer of the epidermis. They may be the result of a previously existing inflammation, disease, or due to an abnormal dryness of the skin. They are found in scarlet fever, eczema, psoriasis, etc. Remember dandruff, and you will not forget what scales look like.

CRUSTS.—Synonyms—Crustae; Scabs; Ger., Krusten.
Crusts are dried masses of exudation. They may consist of blood, serum, pus, fat, and scales of dried skin. The barber should at all times be careful when crusts are seen on the face or scalp, because they often contain germs of a contagious nature. Some of the contagious diseases that have crusts include

13

impetigo, contagiosa, favus, and often syphilis, and a number of others.

ULCERS.—Synonym—Ulcera; Ger., Geschwüre.
Ulcers are due to losses of substance of the skin, caused by disease. They may be of contagious or non-contagious origin.

SCARS.—Synonyms—Cicatrices; Ger., Narben.
Scars are connective tissue new formations, replacing losses of substance, caused by injury, partial or whole destruction of the true skin. A cut with the razor into the true skin will produce a scar, and the deeper the cut the more permanent will be the scar.

INTRODUCTION

Everyone knows that the barber has his ups and downs, the same as those of other trades and professions, and that if he intends to do justice to himself and patron, he must acquaint himself first: with the best method of shaving and cutting hair. Second, he should have a fair knowledge of the appearance of all the contagious diseases with which he may come in contact. Third, he must know the value of antiseptics, which to use, and how to use them, in order to protect himself and his patrons from spreading diseases. The barber comes in contact with various diseases of the skin, some highly contagious, and others not. It is not easy for an inexperienced eye to differentiate a contagious from a non-contagious disease. It is easier to prevent the spread of diseases than it is to cure them. The medical profession makes a distinction between contagious and infectious diseases, but for convenience, the reader may do well to consider these two words as meaning the same. We will now study only those diseases which are of special interest to the barber, either, because they are contagious, or have other scientific or diagnostic value. Syphilis will be explained thoroughly, so as to produce a lasting impression upon the minds of the barbers, and at the same time remind them more strongly of the duties towards their patrons.

SYPHILIS

Synonyms.—Lues Venera; Pox; Bad Disorder; French, Vérole; Italian, Sifilide; Ger., Lustseuche, Krankheit der Franzosen; Swedish, Radezyge.

Syphilis is a chronic, specific, contagious disease, both acquired and transmissible by inheritance, and may produce lesions in any part of the body. The name by which the disease is most often recognized in all languages was first employed by Hieronymus Fracastorius, who, in the year 1521, composed a poem in which a herdsman, named Syphilus, was afflicted with some mysterious malady by the god Apollo, for giving divine honors to the king. The derivation of the word taken from the Greek, was evidently intended by the author to suggest, in no reproachful sense, that the hero of his verses was a simple companion of swine.

Syphilis is most often contracted by sexual intercourse, but may also enter the system by the lips and mouth, through the use of drinking cups and glasses, smoking pipes, by blowing various musical or other instruments, tin horns that are so common around election time, lung testers, that in former years were so frequently seen in saloons and other public places, by kissing, etc. Wet nurses, while nursing syphilitic children, and vice-versa, is another source by which the disease may be carried from one person to another. Syphilitic virus may enter the system by the skin through an abrasion, cut, prick, etc. No part of the skin or mucous membrane is exempt from being inoculated.

Syphilis is divided into three stages, viz.: primary, secondary and tertiary stage.

Primary Stage.

The initial or first lesion of syphilis is the chancre. It marks the place where inoculation has occurred, and where the virus is introduced into the system. The

16

chancre makes its appearance from 10 to 30 days after exposure, and manifests itself most often as a papule, which generally grows larger and harder as time goes on, due to the process of a deep-seated inflammation. The time between the primary lesion and the secondary eruption is generally considered from 30 to 90 days.
Second Stage.

The glands nearest to the point of inoculation become enlarged, and somewhat painful to the touch. The patient will complain of other constitutional symptoms, such as fever, headaches, and pain in the joints. Later an eruption will appear on the skin, which may be universal over the whole, or parts of the body surface. The eruption may appear in the form of macules, papules, pustules, or ulcers. At this time the patient may also complain of sore throat, and of sores in the mouth and nose, and on the tongue. The eyes often become inflamed. While these symptoms go on the hair fall out, which loss is only temporary. There may be a general thinning of the hair, or they may come out in some part more than in others, forming almost nearly bald spots. On the scalp this thinning of hair is most pronounced, but it will also be noticed in the eyebrows and beard. The barber should be on guard when such a condition presents itself to him, but should at the same time not forget that there are other diseases in which the hair fall out, and not look upon every person as being syphilitic in whom such a condition exists.
Third Stage.

Between the second and third stage of syphilis no exact dividing line can be drawn, since the secondary and tertiary symptoms often merge into each other, and while some symptoms which usually occur late in the disease are occasionally among the early manifestations, and some secondary symptoms recur at a late period.

The third stage of syphilis is ascribed to the period in which there appear deep seated swellings called gummata, which often break down, and if not treated, form ulcers. These ulcers terminate in scars, which sometimes will cause unsightly, and permanent disfigurations. Ulcerations may occur on any part of the body. The skin as well as the internal organs may be affected. Paralysis, either of small or large areas, is not uncommon. In some syphilitics the spinal cord may become affected by the disease, which causes a loss of control of the limbs, mostly the lower. When the brain is the seat of a gumma, one-half of the whole body becomes paralyzed, and the patient will have all the symptoms of an apoplectic stroke, and may die during such a period. Insanity is sometimes a sequel of syphilis. Ulcerations of the bones, slight or severe, is another condition sometimes met with in the later stages of syphilis.

The medical profession generally considers that a course of treatment must extend over a period of from two to three years to effect a cure.

WARNING TO THE BARBER

You have heard that syphilis is a contagious disease; that it is chronic in character; that at times it causes destruction of tissue to such an extent that the area involved in regaining its former appearance is out of the question; that such destruction of tissue produces unsightly scars, which sometimes cause great disfiguration, especially if on exposed parts of the body; that such disfigurations are a detriment to the person afflicted, in business transactions, or socially. You have also read that syphilis sometimes produces grave nerve and brain symptoms, insanity, and early death, which facts cannot be impressed too much on the barber's mind. After reading and hearing so much about that dreaded disease, syphilis, the question arises: can a barber knowingly, or through his ignorance or carelessness, expose himself or his patrons to the infection of such a disease, and yet clear his conscience by saying? "I did not know that the man had syphilis whom I shaved." A very flimsy excuse indeed. If a person afflicted with syphilis presents himself to the barber to be shaved or have his hair cut, the barber must be very careful not to prick or cut himself, for fear of contracting the disease. He must never strop the razor he is using on such a person without having it previously well disinfected. If the razor is not disinfected, the strop will be infected, and this careless procedure will be dangerous to others.

RINGWORM

Synonyms.—Tinea tricophytina; Ger., Scherende Flechte.

Ringworm is a contagious disease, and may occur on the scalp, face or body. When on the scalp it is called tinea tonsurans, when on the face, tinea barbae, and when on the body the name tinea circinata is applied to it. The disease is caused by the tricophyton tonsurans fungus, which is a vegetable parasite. The disease is not only a disease of man, but it also frequent in lower animals. Cats, dogs, rabbits, cows, horses, and other animals are liable to it, and have transmitted it to man, and vice-versa. It may also be conveyed through the medium of wearing apparel, towels, toilet articles, etc. Schools, orphan asylums, foundling homes, barber shops, hair dressing and beauty parlors and laundries are common sources.

RINGWORM OF THE SCALP

This disease is mostly found in children. It is transmitted from one child to another, or from lower animals to child, and vice-versa. It begins as a red pimple around a hair, which spreads and becomes a scaly patch of a pale grayish-red color, covered with fine, white scales. This patch widens out, and as the fungi get down into the hair pouches, the hair will show signs of ill nutrition, and have the appearance of being bitten off, are lustreless, and stand in all directions. If an attempt is made to pull them out they often break off below the surface of the skin. Some patches while spreading clear up in the center, others do not. In some cases, patches may take on a more inflammatory nature, and have a different appearance than above described. When such a condition exists, the inflamed patch is somewhat raised, has a more or less boggy appearance, and around the hairs are small pustules. Thick crusts form, and if pressure be made on them, a thick, muco-purulant secretion can readily be ejected.

Ringworm of the scalp is at times very easily cured, but in neglected cases it may persist indefinitely.

RINGWORM OF THE BEARDED REGION

Synonyms.—Tinea sycosis; tinea barbae; barber's itch; Ger., Parasitische Bartfinne.

Ringworm of the bearded region is not met with as frequently as it is on the scalp or body surface. Two distinct types are known. One is superficial, while the other is deep seated and presents a lumpy appearance. The superficial as well as the deep seated variety begins as a slightly scaly, reddish, rounded patch, which has a tendency to spread. The superficial type goes on spreading in the same manner as it started, while the deep seated, after some time, extends down into the deeper layers of the skin, and produces more inflammation. In the superficial variety the hairs and follicles are affected, and the hair can be easily extracted, and others drop out spontaneously. The hair will again grow in, after the disease has subsided.

RINGWORM OF THE GENERAL SURFACE

Ringworm on the general surface or tinea circinata may occur at any age, but children and young adults are more prone to it than old persons. It begins as a small pale-red ,slightly raised scaly spot, the border of which is sharply cut. A spot continues to spread, clearing up in the center and forming a ring. Sometimes these spots do not clear up in the center, and yet continue to spread. Ringworm on the general surface is due to the

21

same fungus as is ringworm of the scalp or bearded region, and is contracted in the same manner. Most cases of ringworm, if treated early, respond readily to treatment.

Ringworm is frequently contracted in unclean, unsanitary barber shops, through the medium of towels and aprons, which are supposed to serve too many patrons before they are discarded, through brushes and combs, razors, tweezers, etc., that are seldom or never sterilized, and last, but not least, through the barber's hands, when only occasionally washed, and probably never disinfected.

IMPETIGO CONTAGIOSA

Impetigo contagiosa is an acute, highly contagious, inflammatory disease of the skin, characterized by the formation of discreet, superficial, flattened, rounded oval vesicles or blebs, and drying to thin yellowish crusts. In most cases the vesicles or blebs contain serum at the beginning, but occasionally their contents are of a mixture of serum and pus. If such a vesicle or bleb is broken, or the skin removed, a moist, red, raw looking surface is exposed. In children the disease is mostly seen to begin around the mouth and nose, and from there spreads to various other parts of the body surface. The disease is generally carried from one child to another, by the hands, slate and lead pencils, various musical instruments that are played by the mouth, toys, and other things that children are in the habit of handling much. At certain times of the year, and in densely populated districts, the disease often becomes epidemic. Adults may contract the disease in the same manner as do children, but in the main, the source of contagion can be traced to the barber shop. This is the disease that is generally known as barber's itch, and is very frequent. The name barber's itch, although wrongly applied to this disease by the barbers, the laity, and by some physicians, is, as stated above, a contagious disease, more so than is ringworm, but is caused by pus inocculation, whereas ringworm is due to a parasite. In impetigo there may be itching, either mild or severe. The patient often complains of a burning sensation. Fresh lesions appear from day to day, and leaving red spots after the vesicles or blebs have dried up and the crusts fallen off. Impetigo contagiosa is most often seen on the face, but may also occur on the scalp, neck, hands or body. If seen early, the disease responds readily to proper treatment, which will save the patient from

23

discontinuing his work, and the annoyance of being stared at by everyone. Persons afflicted with this disease should not be shaved by the barber, unless the necessary precautions are taken. If the rules, how to disinfect the hands and instruments are studied and followed to the letter, there will be little danger of transmitting the disease from one person to another.

FAVUS

Synonyms.—Tinea favosa; crusted ringworm; Ger., Erbgrind.

Favus is a contagious, parasitic disease of the skin, caused by a vegetable parasite. The disease appears in yellow cup-shaped crusts, from a pin's head to a pea in size. At the beginning each crust is pierced by a hair. The disease spreads very slowly, and it may take months before the appearance of the lesions have changed much. Later the crusts unite and form mortar-like masses. The hair within the diseased area have loosened, become brittle, have lost their lustre, break off, and many split longitudinally. The most favorable site for favus is the scalp, but it may attack any part of the body surface. Sometimes the mucous membrane is affected. Favus on the scalp has a more or less characteristic odor, which reminds one of musty straw, and the urine of mice. The young are more liable to contract the disease than do adults. Although favus is seen in adults, it generally has existed for a number of years, and had its beginning while the patient was comparatively young. Favus is not as highly contagious as is ringworm. It is conveyed from one person to another, or from animals, such as dogs, cats, rabbits, cattle or horses, to man. If the disease occurs on the body, in most cases the source of contagion can be traced to the scalp of the same person.

ERYSIPELAS

Synonyms.—The rose; St. Anthony's fire; Ger., Rothlauf; Hautrose; Wundrose.

Erysipelas is a specific inflammatory disease of the skin with constitutional disturbances, such as chills, fever, nausea and sometimes vomiting. The face, and particularly the regions around the nose, are the most common seats of origin. At the beginning of the disease there is a slight redness and swelling, which, while the disease spreads, becomes more and more pronounced. The color will change to a dark red, and the swelling at times is so great as to close both eyes. The border of the redness is sharply defined, and it can be readily seen how far the disease has advanced. The disease often spreads over the whole face and scalp. In some cases blisters form. Delirium may be present when fever is very high. When the disease subsides, the swelling will gradually disappear, and a slight shedding of the horny layer of the skin is noticed. In some cases the hair fall out in great quantities, but will subsequently fill in to the original amount.

Erysipelas may occur at any age, but it is more frequently observed between the ages of twenty and fifty. The cause of erysipelas can often be traced to an injury, such as cuts, pricks, or cracks in the skin, bruises, and in fact anything that injures the skin and produces an opening into which the germ of the disease can readily enter. As a rule, persons with erysipelas do not present themselves at barber shops, but the barber may be called to their homes to shave them. It is advisable in a good natured manner to refuse to shave such persons.

LUPUS VULGARIS

Synonyms.—Lupus; Ger., Fressende Flechte.

The word lupus translated means, a wolf. Lupus is a deep seated inflammation in the skin, producing papules, nodules, and patches, caused by the tubercle bacillus, chronic in course, terminating in ulceration and scarring. The disease is most often seen on the face, and especially on the nose, or its immediate surroundings, but may occur on any part of the body surface. It generally makes its appearance in papules or nodules of a brownish-red or yellowish color, which unite and form a patch. More papules form, the patch enlarges, the old papules or nodules break down and form ulcers, which terminate in scarring. This process may go on for years before an area of one to two inches across is involved. The appearance of the border and the old scarred patch is not unlike that of certain forms of syphilitic lesions, but if the color, the arrangement and hue of the papules, and the slowness of growth are taken into consideration, it will be comparatively easy to make a correct diagnosis. Ringworm is sometimes mistaken for lupus. Lupus leaves scars, ringworm never. The border of lupus consists of papules, whereas ringworm has none. Ringworm spreads rapidly, lupus slowly. The barber should disinfect his hands and instrument well, after shaving a person affected with lupus, and should take all necessary precautions during the time of shaving.

LUPUS ERYTHEMATOSUS

Lupus erythematosus is an inflammatory, chronic disease of the skin, appearing in pinkish or dark-red patches, covered with grayish, or yellowish scales, and most commonly attacking the face. The most favored sites for this affection are the nose and cheeks, ears and scalp. The patches are somewhat elevated, and this is more perceptible at the border line. The scales covering these patches are of a grayish, or yellowish-gray, scant, or in abundance. There may be one or more patches, and from time to time others may appear. They spread, and often two unite and form one. The border of a patch, and the abruptness by which it terminates, produces a striking contrast from the healthy skin surrounding it. Lupus erythematosus is a disease most common between the ages of 16 and 40, but is often seen later than 40, and sometimes before 16. There is at present no absolute certainty as to the cause of this disease. Some authors claim that it is caused by the baccillus of tuberculosis, others hold different views. It will be well for the barber to take the same precautions as he would with lupus vulgaris.

ALOPECIA

Synonyms.—Baldness; Ger., Kahlheit.

The name alopecia is taken from the Greek, meaning a fox. The name was applied to this disease because the fox is prone to baldness. The name alopecia is applied to any kind of baldness, no matter what caused it. It may be due to a constitutional disease, such as syphilis, typhoid fever, erysipelas, old age, disease or injury to nerves, parasitic skin diseases, any of which may cause baldness.

ALOPECIA AREATA

Alopecia Areata is an affliction most often located on the scalp, but may attack any hairy regions on the body. It appears in bald, rounded patches, which at first small and not noticeable to the patient, become larger, the hair fall out, and leave a bright, bald, shining surface. This process may go on until the larger part of the scalp is affected. In exceptional cases the whole scalp may become bald. The hairs at the border of a patch are loose, and can be easily extracted. The skin in and around a patch is not inflamed, nor does it scale. Alopecia areata is caused by a parasite, or may be of neurotic origin. The disease occurs most frequently in persons between the ages of 10 and 30, but may also be found in children younger than 10, and adults older than 30 years of age. Most all cases of this affection take a chronic course. The patches may become covered with a new growth of hair, but this is often of short duration, and the bald area may spread to a larger size than before. While some cases of alopecia areata are contagious and others not, the barber is advised to treat all his patrons afflicted with this disease as if it were of a contagious character, and to take the necessary precautions.

29

SEBORRHOEA

Synonyms.—Stearrhea; Ger., Schmeerfluss; Gneis.

Seborrhoea is a disease of the fat-producing glands of the skin, secreting an abnormal amount of oily substance, or an accumulation of scales or crusts on the skin surface. Two varieties of this disease are known, and are named seborrhoea oleosa, and seborrhoea sica. The former is practically only an excessive oiliness of the skin, the latter is the same, only with an accumulation of scales from the epidermis in addition. These scales are matted together by the oily secretions, and form grayish, dirty, and greasy looking crusts. The disease is most often seen on the scalp and face, and frequently at the junction of the two, and is not of an inflammatory nature. It is most frequently between the ages of 15 and 30, but may occur in children younger than 15 years of age. In the new born it is a common affection, and is generally known by the name, milk crusts.

Some authors claim seborrhoea contagious, but this is not as yet an established fact, only an advanced theory.

ACNE VULGARIS

Synonyms.—Acne; Ger., Akne; Finnen.

Acne is an inflammatory disease of the sebaceous glands, most often of a chronic nature, occurring on the face, shoulders and upper parts of the trunk, and appearing in papules, tubercles and pustules. The disease is common between the ages of 13 and 30. Although the disease may appear on almost any part of the body, yet the face is the most common site. Papules are always present, but they are intermingled with pustules, and often nodules. Comedones (blackheads) are common in acne vulgaris, which are caused by the blocking up of the sebaceous ducts by dried sebaceous secretion. The dark or blackheads on these comedones are due to dust and dirt. Blackheads are most often found in the center of acne papules and pustules, which, when pus is discharged, often leave a stained, pitted scar. These stains will gradually disappear, but the scars will not. Acne vulgaris is not contagious, is met with in barber shops probably more often than any other skin disease, and is very easily recognized.

31

ACNE ROSACEA

Synonyms.—Rosacea; Ger., Kupferrose; Kupferfinne.

Acne rosacea is a chronic disease of the face, which most often makes its appearance on the nose and its immediate surroundings. It is also seen on the forehead and chin, and broadly speaking, is a disease that attacks the middle third of the face. The superficial blood vessels become dilated, giving the area involved a fiery appearance. Papules are present, which often terminate in pustules. From time to time new papules, sometimes nodules spring up, and the disease gradually spreads, involving a greater area. In some of the long standing cases the disease sometimes changes its color from that of bright-red to a blueish hue. It is often stated that the disease is caused by excessive indulgence in alcoholic drinks, but this is a wrong impression, and should be discarded. The disease may be aggravated by dyspepsia, too much drinking of coffee and beverages containing alcohol, but sometimes the cause is obscure. There are some cases in whom the disease has been brought on by the excessive use of alcoholics, but there are others that never drink alcohol in any form. Women are as often affected as are men.

No one should think a person a toper because he has acne rosacia, while he may be right in one case he may be wrong in a number of others. Acne rosacia is not contagious.

DANDRUFF

Dandruff, also called dandriff, is an excessive exfoliation from the horny layer of the epidermis, brought on either by natural dryness or by inflammation of the skin of the scalp, causing an accumulation of scales. These scales are of a white ,or dirty white, or grayish color, dry, or greasy to the touch. There are many diseases in which dandruff is a secondary condition. Seborrhoea, eczema, ringworm and psoriasis are examples. To remove dandruff permanently the disease that causes it must be removed first.

ATROPHY OF THE HAIR

Atrophy (a wasting or innutrition) of the hair is a term employed to cover various abnormal conditions of the hair, manifesting retrogressive changes. These changes may be caused by the invasion of parasites into the hair, or in the immediate surrounding of the hair roots, or any systematic disturbance that causes the nutrition of the hair to be lessened or entirely shut off. The hair become weakened and fragile. Such conditions as stated are found in ringworm, erysipelas, typhoid fever, favus, and numerous other diseases.

SUPERFLUOUS HAIR

This condition may occur on various parts of the skin, but it is only of importance when on exposed surfaces. The face is the most favored locality. The hair are generally grouped on the site of a mole. The treatment for such a condition is the electric needle.

SPLIT HAIR

This is a condition in which the hair are extremely fragile. There are several ways in which this condition is manifested. The hair may split at its free end, along the shaft, and even into the root. In some cases the hair break off when being combed or brushed. This may be barely noticeable, or it may be pronounced. Men with long beards and with long scalp hair are more prone to it. The parts of the hair most often affected are the ends, but the shaft may also be split up for some distance. There are exceptional cases where this splitting occurs along the shaft primarily. In some this splitting is universal, while in others only the hair of cetrain areas are affected. The treatment consists in removing the cause, if this can be determined, by constitutional treatment. Locally the barber can aid towards effecting a cure by frequent shaving of the beard for some time. If the skin is very dry at the affected places, shampooing, and the application of some oily substance thereafter will be of benefit.

RARE DISEASES OF THE HAIR

Some of the rare diseases of the hair that are of little importance to the barber need only mentioning. The beaded heir, in which the hairs contain one, to numerous constrictions along their shafts, which gives them the appearance of a number of spindle shaped beads, placed on a string. The nodose hair, giving the hair the appearance of lice nits being stuck on. In this condition the hairs are very brittle and easily break off at one of the nodules. Some of these diseases seem to be of parasitic origin, but this fact has not as yet been established.

INGROWN HAIR

This condition is caused by too close shaving. The skin being somewhat elastic, is drawn and stretched by the hand of the barber to make shaving easier; this presses the hair more to the surface, and is, while being shaved off, in fact cut below the surface when the skin has receded to its normal position. Another contributary cause is the inflammation produced by shaving.

35

This inflammation, although considered very moderate, is sufficient to cause a swelling of the skin, which partially closes the orifices of the hair follicles over the hair stumps that have been cut off so short. Hair stumps after shaving present a square, or somewhat slant top surface, and while these stumps are growing, sometimes cannot force themselves through the swollen canal orifices, which act as a roof over them, and naturally, will turn and coil up. If this process goes on for some time, an inflamed nodule will make its appearance, which later terminates in an abcess. Opening of this abcess and the removal of the hair is the only treatment.

HAIR SINGEING

The method of treating the hair after being cut by singeing, with the idea of sealing up the ends to prevent the escape of nutrition that should be saved, is a wrong one. Singeing has absolutely no value whatever as a stimulant to make the hair grow, and should rather be considered as a detriment to them. By singeing, the hair stumps are sealed up, which in itself is a worthless procedure, but they are at the same time damaged by the heat, to about an inch, or even more, in addition. From a pecuniary standpoint only is singeing of value, otherwise this practice should be condemned.

THE BARBER HIMSELF

We all must admit that every person has his faults, the barber not excepted. To be faulty is a disgrace in the eyes of the general public. Each person sees the sliver in his neighbor's eye, but will he see the beam in his own? The bad qualities a person may have are spoken of often, whereas the good seldom. When a patron has contracted a disease in a barber shop the people in the whole district are informed about it, but when good, clean treatment is accorded him it will not be interesting news for others.

A barber should protect himself as well as his patrons from contagious diseases. It is not necessary to refuse to shave because a patron is afflicted with such a disease, if the necessary precautions are resorted to. It is criminal to be negligent in this direction. Most diseases contracted in barber shops are spread through the medium of the barber's hands, or his filthy instruments.

When a barber himself is afflicted with a contagious disease it doubles his responsibility towards his patrons. What is he to do? He should wash, and disinfect his hands thoroughly before shaving; he should never place his fingers on the lips, or put them into the patient's mouth; he should be careful not to cut or scratch the skin while shaving, because an abrasion in the skin is the channel through which contagious disease germs are most often transmitted. A styptic should be applied to every cut or scratch immediately after they appear. The barber should not wipe his nose nor use his handkerchief while shaving. A handkerchief is never aseptic while in use; he should not strop his razor on the palms of his hands, neither test its edge on his finger tips, finger nails, or his hair, unless he disinfects it thereafter. It would be criminal negligence for a barber to wet the alum or other styptic with the sputum of his mouth before using it; he should not place his face too close to that of his patron, so as to inhale his, or he your breath; he should never dress wounds or treat

37

other diseases of a contagious nature on his own or other persons, without a thorough disinfection of his hands thereafter; he should never use water from finger-bowls for shaving. While on duty he should have his mind constantly on the dangers to which his patrons are exposed.

The diseases to which a barber should give his full attention, if afflicted himself, are: syphilis, gonorrhoea (clap), soft chancres, veneral warts, and all other veneral diseases, impetigo contagiosa, ringworm, favus, lupus, consumption, and all other tubercular diseases. If the barber is affected with erysipelas he should stay away from his shop until entirely cured.

The barber is advised not to speak to his patrons about the diseases of other patrons, and should not condemn other barbers because some one has contracted a disease at one, or the other's shop. He should bear in mind that some day others may speak of him in the same manner. Would he like it? The barber often comes in contact with persons afflicted with diseases of of the skin, some of which being contagious, others not. At times it will be very difficult for him to differentiate a contagious from a non-contagious disease. In such cases what is he to do? In doubtful cases the barber should, after shaving, not only wash his hands and wipe his razor on a towel, but should wash both, and thoroughly disinfect them thereafter. This being done, there will be little danger of transmitting diseases from one person to another during the time of shaving or cutting hair. It should be the aim of all barbers to have all their instruments, cups, strops, combs, brushes and linens, as much as possible, in an aseptic condition. The barber's chair, and especially its head-rest, should not be greasy, sticky, and all smeared up. The barber must not have cuspidors standing around his shop, that the very sight of them would make any one gag on account of tobacco juice seen all over them, around them, and on the walls of his shop. He should wear clean clothes, and have the fixtures, furniture and floors of his shop clean, and kept clean at all times. The floors should be scrubbed often and at regular intervals. The greasy looking dirt rings which one so often sees around the door knobs and drawer handles of fixtures are certainly not considered by patrons as being ornamental.

SEPSIS

A toxic or putrefactive condition.

ASEPSIS

The meaning of asepsis is, to purify. The word is applied to a condition absolutely free from putrefaction. Aseptic hands, instruments, dressings, etc., are those free from putrefaction.

ANTISEPTICS

The word antiseptic is composed of two words, anti, against, and septic, putrefaction. They are agents that destroy putrefaction.

DISINFECTION

The destroying of disease germs by means of heat, chemic substances, fumigation, or fresh air.

DISINFECTANTS

Agents that destroy disease germs and noxious properties of fermentation and putrefaction.

STERILIZATION

The condition of rendering sterile, infertile, or incapable of reproducing. Sterile hands or instruments are those on which all germs are destroyed, so they cannot reproduce disease.

HOW TO MAKE ANTISEPTIC SOLUTIONS

To make solutions of various strengths it will be necessary to know the drug or chemical that is to be employed, the strength in which it may be used, the amount necessary, and the quantity of the solution to be made. The quantity of the chemical must be in proportion to the quantity of the solution desired. To find the proportions necessary it will be well to study the following rules:

60 grains, minims or drops, make one dram, or one teaspoonful.

8 drams make one ounce, equal to 480 grains or 8 teaspoonfuls.

16 ounces make one pint, or one pound.

2 pints make one quart.

4 quarts make one gallon.

The word grain applies to solid, whereas minims to liquid substances.

The above table is not absolutely correct, because it takes less minims than it does grains, to make one ounce. For all practical purposes, grains and minims should be considered alike, as to their quantity. Certain liquids vary in regard to the size of a drop. A drop of glycerine, syrup or liquid tar is larger and contains more than a drop of alcohol, water, or a drop of an aqueous solution. Liquids may be measured or weighed.

Dry chemicals should never be measured by a teaspoon, but should be weighed when making antiseptic solutions.

A dram contains 60 minims, and is equal to a teaspoonful. A distinction must be made between a teaspoon and a dessertspoon. The latter holds twice the quantity as the former, and this should be kept in mind when making solutions.

When we speak of a 1 to 1,000 solution we mean that one grain or one minim of a certain substance is mixed with or dissolved in 1,000 grains or minims (drops) of another substance. For example: If we intend to make an aqueous antiseptic solution of 1 to 1,000 we must have 1,000 minims of water, to which are added one grain or minim of some chemical. An ounce contains 480 grains or minims (drops). 1,000 drops of water reduced to ounces equals 2 1-12 ounces. A pint contains 16 ounces, and if it requires one grain or minim to 2 1-12 ounces, to make a 1 to 1,000 solution it will take so many grains or minims to the pint as 2 1-12 is contained in 16, which is 7 17-25, or nearly eight grains.

Example:

480 grains or minims make one ounce.

16 ounces make one pint, reduced to minims, gives us

2880
48

7,680 minims, or 7 68-100 equals 7 17-25 grains or minims to make a pint solution of 1 to 1,000 strength.

When we speak of a one % solution, we mean that one grain or drop of a certain substance is mixed with or dissolved in 100 grains or drops of another substance.

To make it clear, let us make a one ounce solution of 1 % strength.

One ounce of water we say contains 480 drops, and if it requires one grain or drop in 100 drops to make a 1 % solution, naturally it will require 4 80-100 grains or drops for a one ounce solution of that strength.

To make a pint solution of 1 % strength, multiply 16 by 4 80-100 equals 76 80-100 grains or drops that are required.

42

For a quart solution multiply 32 (because there are 32 ounces in a quart) by 4 80-100, which will give us 153 60-100 grains or drops required, etc.

If the barber is not already familiar with the rules for making antiseptic solutions, it would be of interest to him to work out several examples, so as to memorize the proportions necessary to make the amount desired of the right strength.

DISINFECTION OF HANDS

Soap and water should be used frequently for washing the hands, and this will for ordinary purposes suffice. When the barber is dealing with contagious diseases he should, after shaving or cutting hair, scrub his hands thoroughly with a brush, in warm water and soap. (An antiseptic soap is preferred.) After washing, rinse in clear water and dip them in an antiseptic solution, or pour the solution over them, rub well, so that the solution will reach into all the folds of the skin. For an antiseptic wash, alcohol pure, or in solution, is the most practicable. Pure grain alcohol is the best, but denatured alcohol that can now be bought at a very much cheaper price than the former, may be used. The only objection to denatured alcohol is, that it is somewhat irritating to the skin. Alcohol may be used undiluted or in solution, varying from twenty-five to fifty per cent. strength. Carbolic acid in solution, from two to five per cent. in water, is a good disinfectant. If a small amount of alcohol is added to the solution it will increase its value as an antiseptic, giving it more penetrating power, and the acid will mix more readily with the water. The objection to carbolic acid is the long lasting odor and the numbness of the fingers and hands that is very often produced by its use.

Formaldehyde (40% solution) may be used as a disinfectant for the hands, in the strength of from one in 100 to one in 1,000 of water. Lysol is another valuable antiseptic, of which one to two per cent. in water is about the strength in which it may be used. Lysol has a very disagreeable odor, which is lasting, and is therefore objectionable. Corrosive sublimate may be used in strength of 1 to 2,000, to 1 to 1,000 of water. A small amount of alcohol added will make it a powerful antiseptic. The objections to the use of corrosive sublimate are: the roughness of the skin of the hands produced by it; instruments are liable to be injured by its corrosive action on them, and the poisonous effect to the system, if frequently employed. There are many other chemicals that may be used as antiseptics, but they are inferior to the above mentioned, or are otherwise objectionable. Remember that the hands must always be washed thoroughly before an antiseptic solution is employed.

DISINFECTION OF FACE AND SCALP

Soap and warm water should always be employed to remove all grease, dried particles of skin, blood, serum, pus, etc., from the face or scalp, before an antiseptic solution is applied. Various solutions may be used to advantage. A twenty-five to fifty per cent. solution of grain alcohol in water, perfumed to suit, makes an efficient and pleasant antiseptic face wash. Witch hazel water, or witch hazel extract, which is generally purchased in drug stores under the name of witch hazel, if not diluted too much, is a good disinfectant. Bayrum not adulterated, is valuable. Witch hazel and bay rum owe their relative antiseptic power to the amount of alcohol they contain. There are many other disinfectants that may be used on the face, but they are no better, or are inferior in value to the above mentioned.

DISINFECTION OF THE RAZOR

For the disinfection of the razor various methods may be employed, but only those that do not injure its cutting edge, or its handle, can be used. One of the most valuable antiseptics for this purpose is alcohol. Undiluted grain alcohol is the best, and should be used. The razor and its handle should be thoroughly washed in warm water and soap so as to remove all particles of skin, blood, serum, pus, etc., rinsed, and boiling water poured over blade. After this is done the whole razor is submerged in alcohol kept in a tray or wide-necked bottle, and left there for several minutes to any time desired. When taking out, dry on a clean towel. The above applies to razors with bone, horn or rubber handles. Some handles of razors are made of metal, which may be disinfected by placing the whole razor into a pan with water, to which a small amount of soda is added, and boiling it for a few minutes, take out and place it in alcohol as mentioned before. A razor thus treated is as aseptic as it can be made. There are many other antiseptics that may be employed, such as carbolic acid, lysol, etc., but they are not as practicable to the barber as is alcohol. Carbolic acid and lysol may be used in 5% strength solution. Formaldehyde, corrosive sublimate and peroxide of hydrogen may spoil the razor.

DISINFECTION OF THE STROP

To disinfect a barber's strop is not very easy to accomplish. In general, strops are somewhat greasy, which prevents aqueous antiseptic solutions from penetrating into the leather. Strong chemicals, and various other non-aqueous antiseptics that will penetrate, are injurious to the leather. If it is desired to clean and disinfect the strop it will be necessary to remove the grease first, which can best be done with a piece of muslin soaked in gasoline, and rubbed over strop until all grease has been removed. After this the strop should be given a light coating of beef tallow previously warmed, so as to penetrate more readily into the leather. This procedure will give the strop its original smoothness as far as it is possible. By placing strops in an air-tight box and fumigating them, is of no value, because the fumes of the chemicals do not penetrate the greasy substance on the strop any more than do aqueous antiseptic solutions. The manner in which a strop may be kept fairly free from putrefactive material, and from germs of contagious diseases, is as follows: A razor should be in good condition before shaving is begun. The razor should not be stropped during the time of shaving. If it is found to give out before shaving is completed, a second one should be resorted to, unless the first one is thoroughly disinfected before it is stropped. The above method will prevent blood, serum, pus, putrefactive material, germs and other dangerous particles from being smeared onto the strop and infecting it.

48

DISINFECTION OF CUP AND BRUSH

Cups should be thoroughly washed in warm water and soap, placed in boiling hot water, or boiling hot water poured over them slowly, to prevent cracking.

Shaving brushes should be washed in warm water and soap, rinsed, the water pressed out with a clean towel, and dipped in alcohol. The superfluous alcohol may be pressed out, and the brush placed into the cup. If brush is supplied with a metallic handle, both may be disinfected as above stated. If the brush has a handle made of wood or other material, and enameled, it should never be used when dealing with contagious diseases. In such cases make the lather in the cup, lay the brush aside, and apply the lather to the face with your fingers. The cup can easily be disinfected, but not so the enameled handle of the brush, because boiling water will not only injure the brush, but also the enamel of the handle, and if alcohol is used it will surely destroy the latter.

DISINFECTION OF COMBS

Combs, if made of bone, horn, or rubber, should be scrubbed well with a brush in warm water and soap, rinsed and laid in alcohol, or alcohol applied to them.

Combs made of metal may be disinfected as above mentioned, or they may be boiled in water for about five to ten minutes.

DISINFECTION OF HAIR BRUSHES

The hair brush is probably one of the barber's most used article to which the least attention is given in re-

49

gard to its disinfection, and is also one of the hardest to disinfect, on account of its peculiar construction.

The handles and backs of hair brushes are generally made of rubber, metal, celluloid, or wood, enameled or painted, or varnished. Brushes should be washed frequently in warm water and some antiseptic soap. If handles and backs of brushes are made of rubber, metal or celluloid, alcohol may be used as a disinfectant, either pure or diluted, after being washed. If enameled, painted or varnished, no alcohol should be used. A thorough cleaning of such hair brushes can be accomplished by the use of gasoline, which will remove all greasy particles that may have adhered to the brush, and if soap and warm water are used thereafter it will render the brush fairly aseptic.

DISINFECTION OF FORCEPS AND TWEEZERS

Forceps, tweezers and other metallic instruments should be disinfected by boiling, each and every time after they have been used, and just before being used, wipe them with a little absorbent cotton soaked with alcohol.

DISINFECTION OF TOWELS, APRONS, LINENS

These are best disinfected by boiling in soap water. No antiseptic solutions are required thereafter.

VIBRATORY MASSAGE

Massage machines are at present comparatively rare in barber shops, and this may be the reason that they are so often used indiscriminately as to their value, or the harm they may produce. The more they will be employed, the more will the advantages and disadvantages be studied. Most barbers of today use them not for the physiological value that may be obtained by them, but only for the psychological effect they produce on patrons. In common words, it is a machine, and at present used in a machinelike manner. These machines are of value in selected cases, where stimulation of the skin is required, and where such stimulation is not indicated, their use does harm.

DISINFECTION OF VIBRATODES

Vibratodes are attachments, some of which are made of soft, others of hard rubber, that come in actual contact with the skin during the time of massering. The most frequently used are those made of soft rubber, and are bell-shaped. Those made of hard rubber are more painful to the patient. The misuse of the vibratodes by some barbers lies in the unscrupulous and ignorant manner in which they use them. They attach them to the handle of the machine all right, and also may know how the machine is started and stopped, but they seldom or never think of taking them off for disinfection. Vibratodes must be detached after each treatment, washed and disinfected. Those made of soft rubber can be boiled in water from five to ten minutes. Soft rubber stands boiling fairly well, although in time is inclined to soften. Another good method by which

51

the soft, as well as the hard rubber vibratodes can be disinfected, is to wash them thoroughly in warm water and germicidal soap, rinse, dry, and place them in a dish containing alcohol, for several minutes. After that they are ready for use.

STYPTICS

Styptics are agents that arrest bleeding. Some of the styptics employed by barbers are: Alum in lump, powder, or in solution, powdered burned alum, the styptic pencil, sugar of lead, sulphate of zinc and others. Alum in lump form must never be used to arrest bleeding by any barber. The reason for this is, that sa a rule lump alum is allowed to lie around on the shelves exposed, handled freely by the septic hands of the barber, and then is applied to a bleeding surface. Blood, serum and germs adhere to it, and the next patron gets them, commonly speaking, rubbed into himself. As a barber, would you willingly expose yourself to such a treatment, knowing that the person previously shaved, and on whom lump alum has been used, had syphilis or another contagious disease? Is the barber so sure that the person he is shaving has no contagious disease, and that lump alum can be used on him without endangering others to be shaved thereafter?

Some barbers of today have discovered a new plan to sidetrack the eyes of the inspectors of the state licensing board in regard to the use of alum, by placing it in their coat pockets, to be used at will. By such a practice the barber not only hides his own ignorance, but preserves disease germs for the next patron. Don't do that. The use of lump alum is against the Wisconsin State laws for barbers, against the rules of hygiene, and against common sense. There is no reason for its employment, except stubbornness, or ignorance. If you are still using lump alum, throw it away before you make some one miserable for his lifetime, with one or another dreadful disease. Alum in powdered or liquid form is the best, cleanest, and safest styptic, if properly used. A clean toothpick, moistened with water, dipped into the powdered alum, and applied to a cut, is very practicable. Alum in solution may be applied in a similar manner, with a little absorbent cotton wound around one end of the toothpick. A toothpick should never be used a second time. An ordinary medicine dropper will also answer the purpose.

The styptic pencil employed so frequently in former years has, we are glad to say, been discarded, and we hope that it will never again make its appearance in barber shops.

Sugar of lead and sulphate of zinc may be employed as styptics in solutions of from three to five per cent. in distilled water.

FACE FOMENTATIONS

The practice of applying wet, hot towels before or after shaving have their advantage and disadvantage. When the skin is somewhat irritable, red and inflamed after shaving, fomentations of wet, hot towels produce a soothing effect, and are very agreeable to the person shaved, but their disadvantage lies in the inhalation of the steam produced by them, which causes a congestion of the mucous membrane of the nose, making it more sensitive to the effects of cold, and giving the nose a feeling as being stuffed up. You often have heard people say that they caught a cold in their nose, which many times if traced, would be found due to hot fomentations. Wet, cold towels, applied to the face after shaving will have an opposite effect on the mucous membrane, but they will not be agreeable to the person shaved. For washing off the soap from the face after shaving, it will be best to use water at a temperature of about 60 degrees.

The towels should be discarded after fomentations are made, and must never be used on other persons without being previously boiled. The practice to lay such towels on marble slabs or shelves, or let them lie around on wash basins to await the next customer, should be condemned. Use a clean towel for every person, or none at all. By applying wet, hot fomentations to the face before shaving, the blood supply of the skin is increased, which makes the ground more fertile for the absorption of disease germs, and is therefore not recommended.

DUSTING POWDER

There is not much to be said about dusting powders. Each barber may use the one he prefers. Dusting powders should never be applied with powder puffs, or rubbed into the skin by the barber's hands. A sprinkling device may be considered the most practicable, and also the most sanitary. Lump magnesia should never be used.

BATHS

Bathtubs must be cleansed after each bath. Wash soda added to the water when cleaning bathtubs is of service. Fresh, clean towels must be furnished for each bath, and the towels should never be dried and used a second time without previous boiling. The barber should not forget to look after the combs and hair brushes of his bathrooms, and should not forget to keep them clean. The bath brush so often seen in barber shop bathrooms is not sanitary, and it probably would be better if it were discarded.

ANTISEPTIC SOAPS

Some of the antiseptic-germicidal soaps that are of value for disinfection for the barber's hands and his instruments are:

Corrosive sublimate soap ½%.
Lysol soap 5 to 10%.
Carbolic acid and glycerine soap 5%.
Formaldehyde soap.
Creolin soap 5%.
Green soap.

Corrosive sublimate soap is a good antiseptic, germicidal and odorless soap.

Carbolic acid and lysol soaps are valuable, but leave a very disagreeable and lasting odor.

Formaldehyde soap may be used. It has a pungent odor which is not lasting.

Green soap, which can be bought at every drug store, may be considered as the best all round soap for the barber. It is of a semi-solid consistency, has no disagreeable odor, and is not expensive.

CONDEMNED RELICS OF THE OLD-TIME BARBER SHOP

Under this heading are mentioned such articles that were formerly used in barber shops and considered at one time or another a necessity, but have been discarded by most barbers as unhygienic, and disease-carrying accessories. They include finger bowls, powder puffs, lump magnesia, lump alum, and the styptic pencil.

While all of the above articles have been fully discussed in other parts of this book, nevertheless, it cannot be impressed too strongly on the mind of every barber, that such articles must never be used. At the present time we have other articles that accomplish the same usefulness, and which are more sanitary at the same time.

58

QUESTIONS THAT WILL AID THE APPRENTICE IN HIS FINAL EXAMINATION

1 Give the name of the most external layer of the skin.

2 State whether the epidermis has blood supply or not?

3 Into which layer of the skin must you cut to produce bleeding?

4 Give the name of the glands that produce perspiration.

5 Give the name of the glands that produce the oiliness of the skin.

6 Name the two chief varieties of blood vessels.

7 Which are the most superficially located blood vessels, the veins or the arteries?

8 Is there any difference in the color of the blood of arteries, from that of veins? Explain.

9 In former years when cupping was practiced by the barbers, what kind of blood was extracted, venous or arterial?

10 In drawing off blood from the skin by cupping it is often said that only the bad blood is drawn. What is your opinion?

11 What furnishes the nutrition to the hair?

12 Describe the functions of the skin.

13 Give an example of a macule.

14 What is the common name for papule?

15 What do vesicles contain?

16 What do pustules contain?

17 From which layer of the skin are scales produced?

18 What are scales?

19 Name one disease of the skin in which scales are produced.

20 What may cause the formation of scales?

21 Give substances that may enter into the composition of a crust.

22 Name one contagious disease in which you expect to find crusts.

23 A cut deep into the skin after being healed up, results in what?

24 Is a scar a permanent disfiguration?

25 Give the common name for syphilis.

26 How may a barber contract syphilis from a person while shaving him?

27 Is syphilis a contagious disease?

28 Is syphilis a chronic disease or not?

29 Name as many ways as you can how syphilis may
    be contracted.

30 What causes ringworm?

31 Is ringworm contagious or not?

32 At what ages do we most often find ringworm on
    the scalp?

33 Ringworm of the bearded region is most common
    between what ages?

34 Name some animals that are prone to ringworm.

35 What appearance do the hair present in ringworm
    of the beard or scalp?

36 Describe the spreading of a patch of ringworm.

37 By what commonly used name is ringworm best
    known?

38 How may ringworm be contracted in barber
    shops?

39 What causes impetigo contagiosa?

40 State whether impetigo contagiosa is highly, feeb-
    ly, or not contagious at all.

41 Can impetigo contagiosa be contracted in barber
    shops?

42 How may impetigo contagiosa be contracted in
    barber shops? State fully.

43 Is impetigo contagiosa often contracted in barber shops?

44 What in your opinion is the cause that so many persons contract impetigo contagiosa in barber shops? State fully.

45 If you were obliged to shave a person afflicted with impetigo contagiosa on the face, how would you proceed?

46 What would you do immediately after shaving a person with impetigo contagiosa?

47 At about what age would you expect to find favus most often?

48 Is favus a contagious disease or not?

49 What causes favus?

50 On what part of the body do we most often see favus?

51 Do we have crust formation in favus?

52 From what animals is favus often contracted?

53 Is Erysipelas contagious?

54 Supposing a person with erysipelas presents himself at your shop for a shave, what would you do?

55 Give the most favored locality for erysipelas.

56 If you are not certain that a case of alopecia areata is contagious or not, and yet you intend to shave or cut hair, what are you to do?

57 Name most favored locality for alopecia areata.

58 What is destroyed in alopecia areata?

59 Describe a patch of alopecia areata.

60 Is acne contagious or not?

61 Which is the most favored locality for acne?

62 How are blackheads caused, and by what?

63 Is acne rosacea always caused by the excessive use of alcoholics?

64 What value, if any, is there in hair singeing?

65 What would you advise for split hair?

66 From which layer of the skin is dandruff produced?

67 Will an inflammation of the skin of the scalp cause dandruff or not?

68 Suppose a person has contracted a contagious disease in a barber shop, to what in your opinion would you attribute the cause?

69 What is sepsis?

70 What do you understand by the word asepsis?

71 Antiseptics, what are they?

72 Explain the meaning of disinfection.

73 What are disinfectants?

74 How would you disinfect your hands?

75 Why should you disinfect your hands after shaving some one with a contagious disease?

63

76 How should your hands be treated before you apply an antiseptic on them?

77 Which in your opinion is the best disinfectant for the barber's hands?

78 Mention two disinfectants for the hands, and how employed.

79 Name two disinfectants for the face and how employed.

80 Disinfect a razor with a bone, horn or rubber handle.

81 Disinfect a razor with a metallic handle.

82 How would you treat a razor before you disinfect it?

83 How can a strop be made fairly aseptic?

84 What value, if any, has fumigation as a disinfectant for the strop?

85 How would you disinfect a shaving cup?

86 How would you disinfect a shaving brush?

87 Supposing a person with a contagious disease presents himself for a shave, how would you make the soap lather, and how should you apply it to the face?

88 Give a method for disinfection of combs.

89 State how you would disinfect a hair brush.

90 How would you disinfect forceps and tweezers?

91 How often do you think it necessary to disinfect forceps and tweezers?

92 Give the only good method for disinfection of towels, aprons and other linens used in barber shops.

93 What is your object in giving vibratory massage?

94 For what conditions of the skin is vibratory massage indicated?

95 How often must vibratodes be disinfected?

96 Name the styptic that you would use to arrest bleeding.

97 How would you arrest bleeding? State fully.

98 What is your opinion of the use of lump alum?

99 Why should lump alum not be used to arrest bleeding?

100 In what forms may alum be used to arrest bleeding?

101 Explain how you would use powdered alum?

102 How would you apply alum in solution?

103 Give your opinion as to the advantage or disadvantage of the styptic pencil.

104 What are antiseptic solutions used for?

105 How many grains of a chemical does it take to a pint of water, to make a solution of 1 to 1,000 strength?

106 How many grains of a chemical to a quart of water to make a solution of 1 to 2,000 strength?

107 Approximately, how many teaspoonfuls of carbolic acid are needed to a gallon of water to make a solution of 1 to 500 strength?

108 How many ounces of alcohol are necessary for a pint solution of 25% strength?

109 Supposing you had a pint bottle in which you wanted to make an alcoholic solution of a 25% strength, and had nothing to measure with, how much alcohol, and how much water would you put into the bottle?

110 Make an ounce of a 2% carbolic solution.

111 Figure out correctly the amount of a chemical needed to make a pint solution of a 3% strength.

112 How do you apply dusting powders to the face?

NOTICE

The "Progressive Barber" can be purchased from all leading barber supply dealers or direct from the secretary of The Wisconsin State Barbers' Board, Milwaukee, Wis., for the price of $1.00.

INDEX

Page

A

68

E

F

H

69